The Complete Mediterranean Breakfast Cookbook

Super Tasty Mediterranean Breakfast Recipes for a healthy lifestyle

Carlo Montesanti

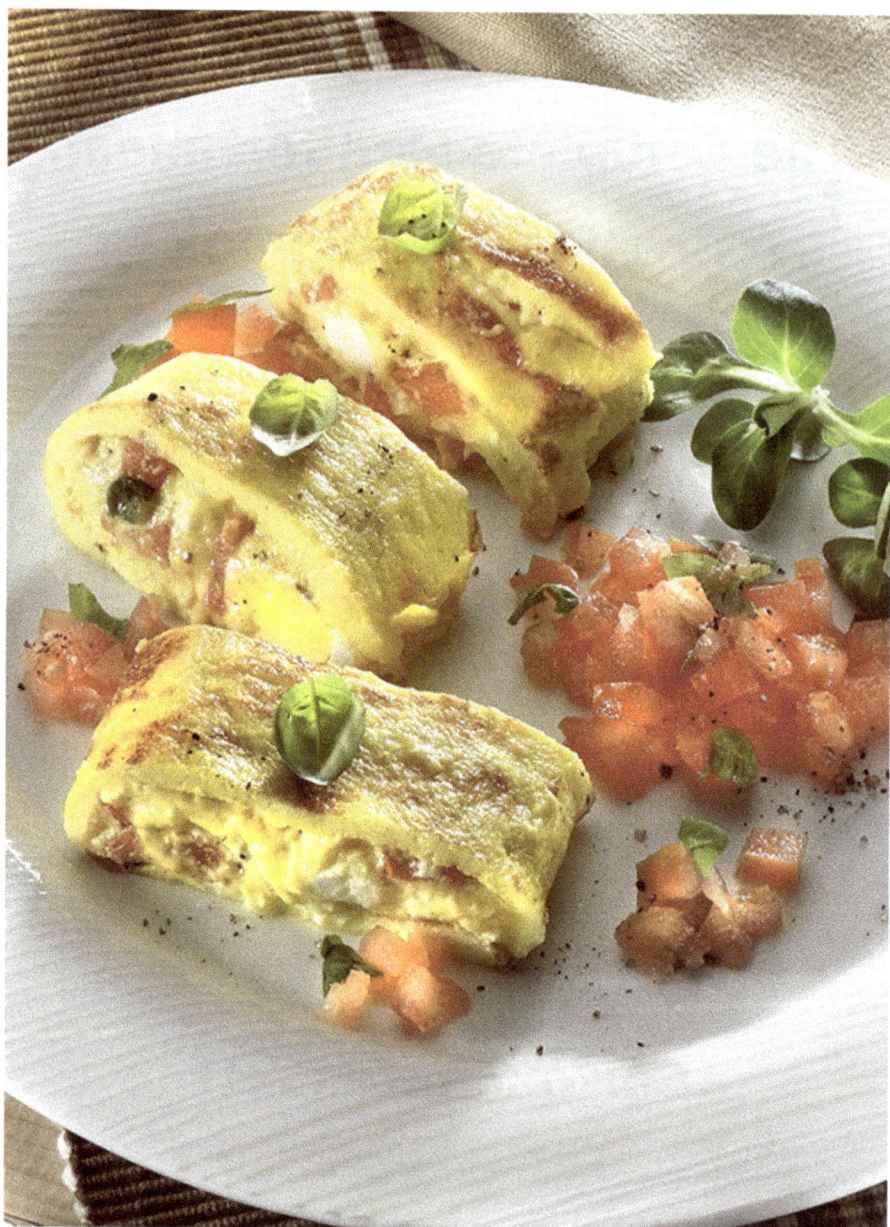

Table of Contents

Green Tart Smoothie

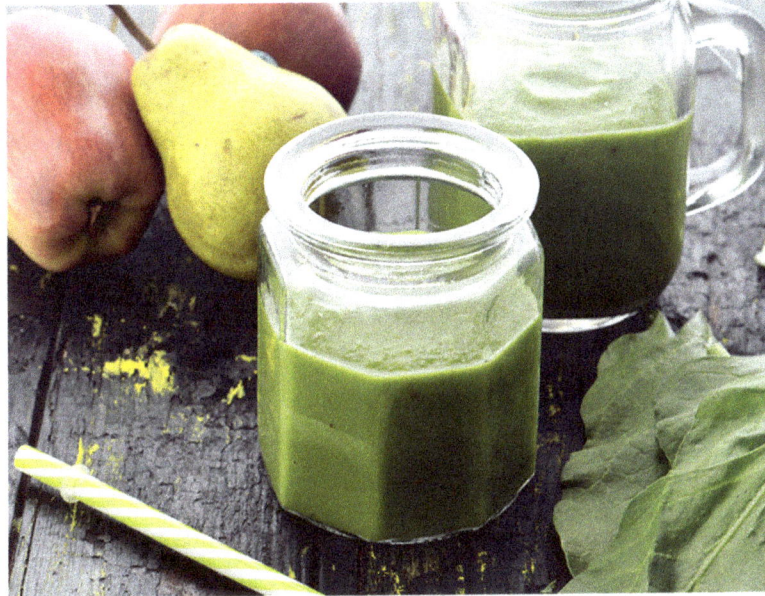

Prep Time: 5 min

Cook Time: 5 min

Serve: 1

Ingredients:

- 2 cups fresh kale
- 1 cup water
- 2 large stalks of celery, chopped
- ½ cucumber, chopped
- 1/3 grapefruit

- 1 cup frozen pineapple

Directions:

1. Blend kale and water until smooth. Add remaining ingredients, and blend until smooth. Enjoy!

Coconut Milk Smoothie

Prep Time: 10 min

Cook Time: 0 min

Serve: 1

Ingredients:

- 1 1/2 cups coconut milk
- 1 frozen banana
- 2 cups raw baby spinach

Directions:

1. Add everything to a food processor. Blend the ingredients well until smooth. Refrigerate until chilled enough. Serve with your favorite garnish.

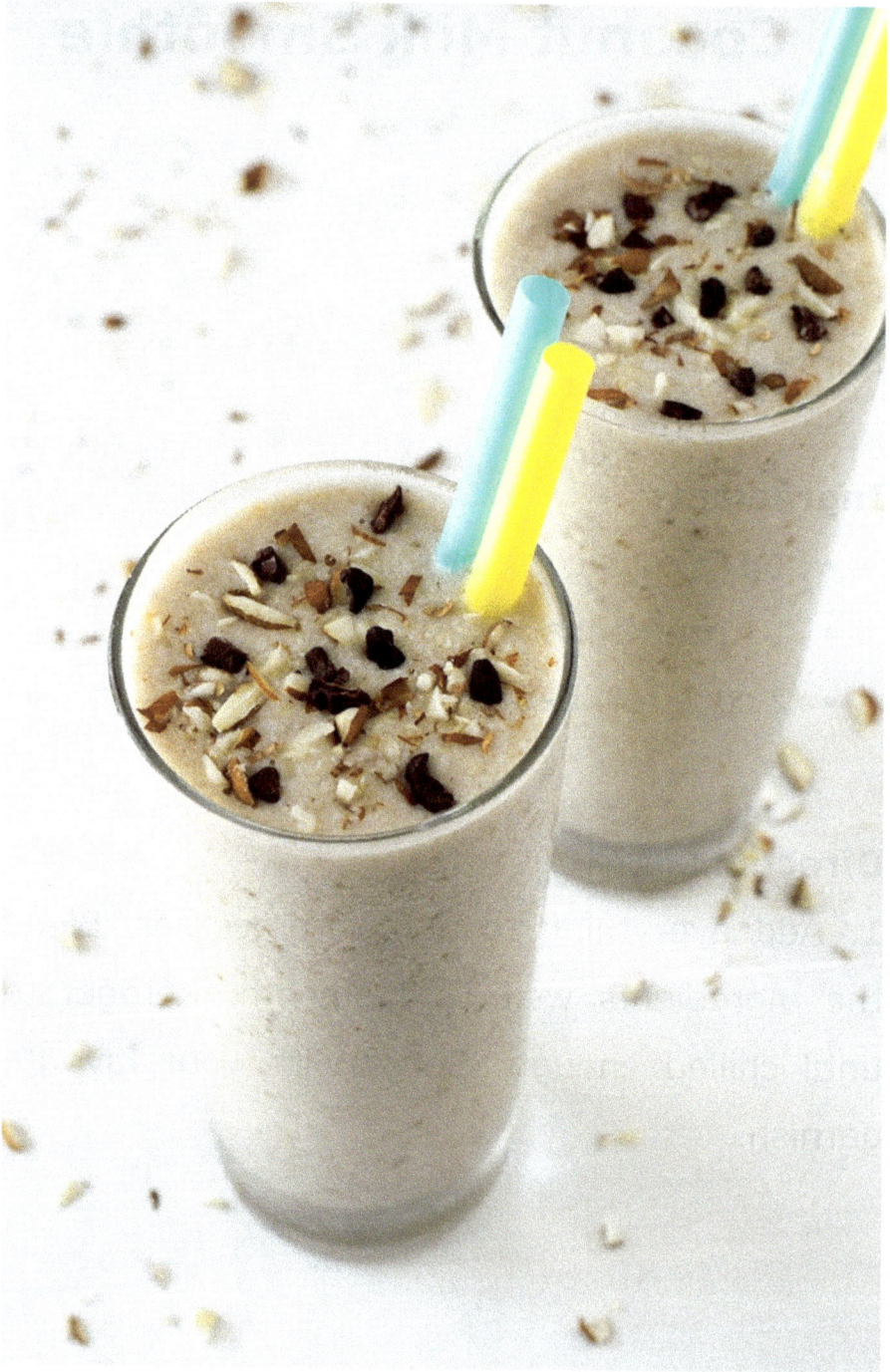

Creamy Strawberry Smoothie

Prep Time: 10 min

Cook Time: 0 min

Serve: 1

Ingredients:

- 1 banana
- 1/2 cup frozen strawberries and 1/2 cup mango
- 1/2 cup Greek yogurt
- 1/4 cup coconut milk
- 1/4 tsp. turmeric
- 1/4 tsp. ginger
- 1 tbsp. honey

Directions:

1. Add everything to a food processor. Blend the ingredients well until smooth.

2. Refrigerate until chilled enough. Serve with your favorite garnish

Alkaline Blueberry Spelt Pancakes

Prep Time: 6 min

Cook Time: 20 min

Serve: 3

Ingredients:

- 2 cups Spelt Flour
- 1 cup Milk and
- 1/2 cup Alkaline Water
- 2 tbsps. Grapeseed Oil
- 1/2 cup Agave
- 1/2 cup Blueberries
- 1/4 tsp. Sea Moss

Directions:

1. Mix the spelt flour, agave, grapeseed oil, hemp seeds, and the sea moss in a bowl. Add in

1 cup of hemp milk and alkaline water to the mixture, until you get the consistency mixture you like.

2. Crimp the blueberries into the batter. Heat the skillet to moderate heat then lightly coat it with the grapeseed oil.

3. Pour the batter into the skillet then let them cook for approximately 5 minutes on every side. Serve and Enjoy.

Alkaline Blueberry Muffins

Prep Time: 5 min

Cook Time: 20 min

Serve: 3

Ingredients:

- 1 cup Coconut Milk
- 3/4 cup Spelt Flour
- 3/4 Teff Flour
- 1/2 cup Blueberries
- 1/3 cup Agave
- 1/4 cup Sea Moss Gel
- 1/2 tsp. Sea Salt Grapeseed Oil

Directions:

1. Adjust the temperature of the oven to 365 degrees. Grease 6 regular-size muffin cups with muffin liners.

2. In a bowl, mix sea salt, sea moss, agave, coconut milk, and flour gel until they are properly blended. You then crimp in blueberries.

3. Coat the muffin pan lightly with the grapeseed oil. Pour in the muffin batter.

4. Bake for at least 30 minutes until it turns golden brown.

Crunchy Quinoa Meal

Prep Time: 5 min

Cook time: 25 min

Serve: 2

Ingredients:

- 3 cups coconut milk
- 1 cup rinsed quinoa
- 1/8 tsp. ground cinnamon
- 1 cup raspberry
- 1/2 cup chopped coconuts

Directions:

1. In a saucepan, pour milk and bring to a boil over moderate heat. Add the quinoa to the milk and then bring it to a boil once more.

2. You then let it simmer for at least 15 minutes on medium heat until the milk is reduced. Stir in the cinnamon then mix properly.

3. Cover it then cook for 8 minutes until the milk is completely absorbed. Add the raspberry and cook the meal for 30 seconds. Serve and enjoy.

Coconut Pancakes

Prep Time: 5 min

Cook Time: 15 min

Serve: 4

Ingredients:

- 1 cup coconut flour
- 2 tbsps. arrowroot powder
- 1 tsp. baking powder
- 1 cup coconut milk
- 3 tbsps. coconut oil

Directions:

1. In a medium container, mix in all the dry ingredients. Add the coconut milk and 2 tbsps. of the coconut oil then mix properly.

2. In a skillet, let melt 1 tsp. of coconut oil. Pour a ladle of the batter into the skillet then

swirl the pan to spread the batter evenly into a smooth pancake.

3. Cook it for like 3 minutes on medium heat until it becomes firm. Turn the pancake to the other side then cook it for another 2 minutes until it turns golden brown.

4. Cook the remaining pancakes in the same process. Serve.

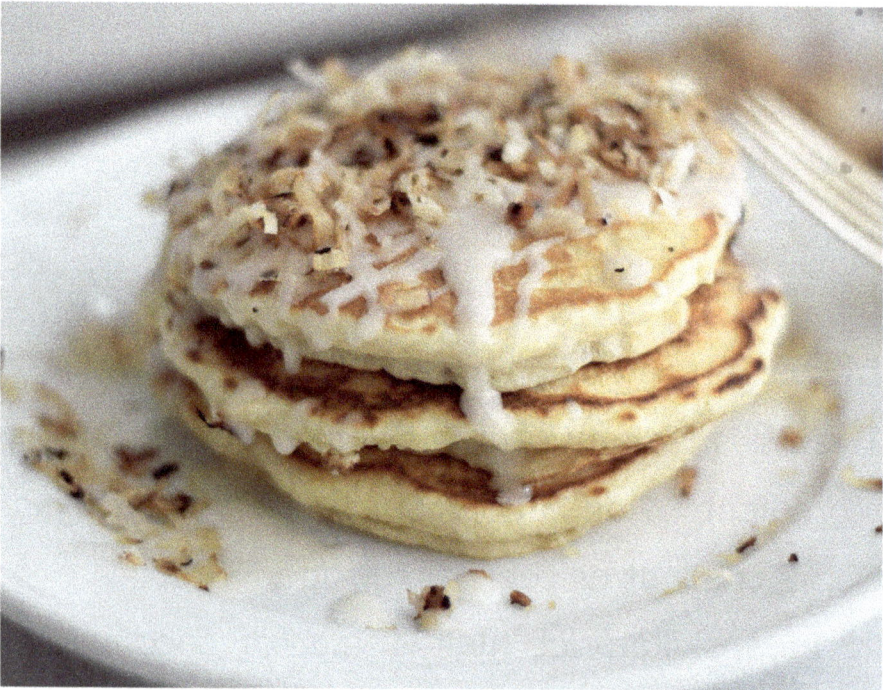

Quinoa Porridge

Prep Time: 5 min

Cook Time: 25 min

Serve: 2

Ingredients:

- 2 cups coconut milk
- 1 cup rinsed quinoa
- 1/8 tsp. ground cinnamon
- 1 cup fresh blueberries

Directions:

1. In a saucepan, boil the coconut milk over high heat. Add the quinoa to the milk then bring the mixture to a boil.

2. You then let it simmer for 15 minutes on medium heat until the milk is reduces. Add the cinnamon then mix it properly in the saucepan.

3. Cover the saucepan and cook for at least 8 minutes until milk is completely absorbed. Add

in the blueberries then cook for 30 more seconds. Serve.

Banana Barley Porridge

Prep Time: 15 min

Cook Time: 5 min

Serve: 2

Ingredients:

- 1 cup divided unsweetened coconut milk
- 1 small peeled and sliced banana
- 1/2 cup barley
- 3 drops liquid stevia
- 1/4 cup chopped coconuts

Directions:

1. In a bowl, properly mix barley with half of the coconut milk and stevia. Cover the mixing bowl then refrigerate for about 6 hours.

2. In a saucepan, mix the barley mixture with coconut milk.

3. Cook for about 5 minutes on moderate heat. Then top it with the chopped coconuts and the banana slices. Serve.

Zucchini Muffins

Prep time: 10 min

Cook time: 25 min

Serve: 16

Ingredients:

- 1 tbsp. ground flaxseed
- 3 tbsps. alkaline water
- 1/4 cup walnut butter
- 3 medium over-ripe bananas
- 2 small grated zucchinis
- 1/2 cup coconut milk
- 1 tsp. vanilla extract
- 2 cups coconut flour
- 1 tbsp. baking powder
- 1 tsp. cinnamon
-
- 1/4 tsp. sea salt

Directions:

1. Tune the temperature of your oven to 375ºF. Grease the muffin tray with the cooking spray.

2. In a bowl, mix the flaxseed with water. In a glass bowl, mash the bananas then stir in the remaining ingredients.

3. Properly mix and then divide the mixture into the muffin tray. Bake it for 25 minutes. Serve.

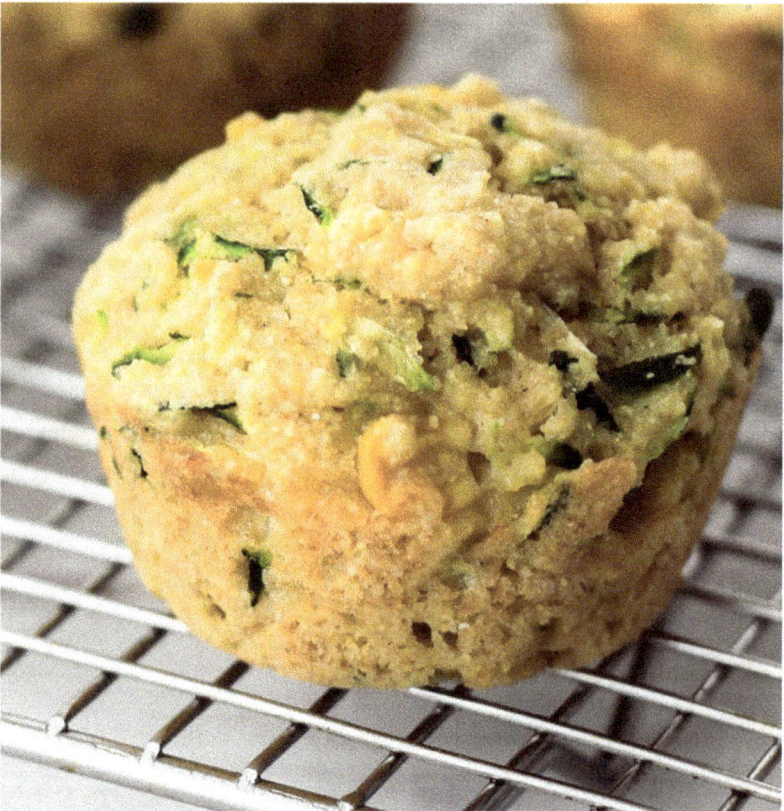

Millet Porridge

Prep Time: 10 min

Cook Time: 20 min

Ingredients:

Serve: 2

- Sea salt
- 1 tbsp. finely chopped coconuts
- 1/2 cup unsweetened coconut milk
- 1/2 cup rinsed and drained millet
- 1-1/2 cups alkaline water
- 3 drops liquid stevia

Directions:

1. Sauté the millet in a non-stick skillet for about 3 minutes. Add salt and water then stir. Let the meal boil then reduce the amount of heat.

2. Cook for 15 minutes then add the remaining ingredients. Stir. Cook the meal for 4 extra

minutes. Serve the meal with toping of the chopped nuts.

Jackfruit Vegetable Fry

Prep Time: 5 min

Cook Time: 5 min

Serve: 6

Ingredients:

- 2 finely chopped small onions
- 2 cups finely chopped cherry tomatoes
- 1/8 tsp. ground turmeric
- 1 tbsp. olive oil
- 2 seeded and chopped red bell peppers
- 3 cups seeded and chopped firm jackfruit
- 1/8 tsp. cayenne pepper
- 2 tbsps. chopped fresh basil leaves
- Salt

Directions:

1. In a greased skillet, sauté the onions and bell peppers for about 5 minutes. Add the tomatoes then stir.

2. Cook for 2 minutes. Then add the jackfruit, cayenne pepper, salt, and turmeric. Cook for about 8 minutes.

2. Garnish the meal with basil leaves. Serve warm.

Zucchini Pancakes

Prep Time: 15 min

Cook Time: 8 min

Serve: 8

Ingredients:

- 12 tbsps. alkaline water
- 6 large grated zucchinis
- Sea salt
- 4 tbsps. ground Flax Seeds
- 2 tsps. olive oil
- 2 finely chopped jalapeño peppers
- 1/2 cup finely chopped scallions

Directions:

1. In a bowl, mix water and the flax seeds then set it aside.

2. Pour oil in a large non-stick skillet then heat it on medium heat.

3. The add the black pepper, salt, and zucchini. Cook for 3 minutes then transfer the zucchini into a large bowl.

4. Add the flax seed and the scallion's mixture then properly mix it. Preheat a grill then grease it lightly with the cooking spray. Pour 1/4 of the zucchini mixture into skillet then cook for 3 minutes. Flip the side carefully then cook for 2 more minutes.

4. Repeat the procedure with the remaining mixture in batches. Serve.

Squash Hash

Prep Time: 2 min

Cook Time: 10 min

Serve: 2

Ingredients:

- 1 tsp. onion powder
- 1/2 cup finely chopped onion
- 2 cups spaghetti squash
- 1/2 tsp. sea salt

Directions:

1. Using paper towels, squeeze extra moisture from spaghetti squash. Place the squash into a bowl then add the salt, onion, and the onion powder. Stir properly to mix them.

2. Spray a non-stick cooking skillet with cooking spray then place it over moderate heat. Add the

spaghetti squash to pan. Cook the squash for about 5 minutes.

3. Flip the hash browns using a spatula. Cook for 5 minutes until the desired crispness is reached. Serve.

Pumpkin Spice Quinoa

Prep Time: 10 min

Cook Time: 0 min

Serve: 2

Ingredients:

- 1 cup cooked quinoa
- 1 cup unsweetened coconut milk
- 1 large mashed banana
- 1/4 cup pumpkin puree
- 1 tsp. pumpkin spice
- 2 tsps. chia seeds

Directions:

1. In a container, mix all the ingredients. Seal the lid then shake the container properly to mix. Refrigerate overnight.

2. Serve.

Sweet Cashew Cheese Spread

Prep Time: 5 min

Cook Time: 5 min

Serve: 10

Ingredients:

- Stevia (5 drops)
- Cashews (2 cups, raw)
- Water (1/2 cup)

Directions:

1. Soak the cashews overnight in water. Next, drain the excess water then transfer cashews to a food processor.

2. Add in the stevia and the water. Process until smooth.

3. Serve chilled. Enjoy.

Mini Zucchini Bites

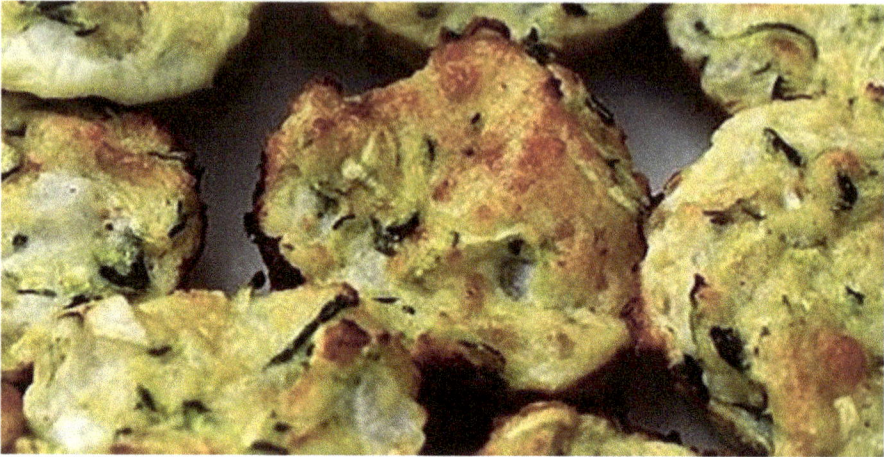

Prep Time: 10 min

Cook Time: 10 minutes

S**erve**: 6

Ingredients:

- 1 zucchini, cut into thick circles
- 3 cherry tomatoes, halved
- 1 tsp. chives, chopped
- 1/2 cup parmesan cheese plus
- Salt and pepper to taste

Directions:

1. Preheat the oven to 390 degrees F. Add wax paper on a baking sheet. Arrange the zucchini pieces.

2. Add the cherry halves on each zucchini slice. Add parmesan cheese, chives, and sprinkle with salt and pepper.

3. Bake for 10 minutes. Serve.

Beef with broccoli on cauliflower rice

Prep Time: 5 min

Cook Time: 15 min

Serve: 2

Ingredients:

- 1 lb. raw beef round steak, cut into strips.
- 1 Tbsp + 2 tsp low sodium soy sauce
- 1 Splenda packet
- ½ C water
- 1 ½ C broccoli florets
- 1 tsp sesame or olive oil
- 2 Cups cooked, grated cauliflower or frozen riced cauliflower

Directions:

1. Stir steak with soy sauce and let sit about 15 minutes. Heat oil over medium-high heat then stir fry beef for 3-5 minutes or until browned. Remove from pan.

2. Place broccoli, Splenda and water. Cook for 5 minutes or until broccoli start to turn tender, stirring sometimes. Add beef back in and heat up thoroughly.

3. Serve the dish with cauliflower rice.

Asparagus & crabmeat frittata

Prep Time: 5 min

Cook Time: 15 min

Serve: 4

Ingredients:

- 2½ tbsp extra virgin olive oil
- plus 2 lbs. asparagus
- 1 tsp salt
- 1 ½ tsp black pepper
- 2 tsp sweet paprika
- 1 lb. lump crabmeat
- 1 tbsp finely cut chives
- ¼ cup basil chopped
- 4 cups liquid egg substitute

Directions:

1. Deter the tough ends of the asparagus and cut it into bite-sized pieces. Preheat an oven to 375°F.

2. In a 12-Inch to a 14-inch oven-proof, non-stick skillet, warm the olive oil and sweat the asparagus until tender. Season with pepper, paprika, and salt.

3. In a mixing bowl, add the chives, crab and basil meat.

4. Pour in the liquid egg substitute and mix until combined.

5. Pour the crab and egg mixture into the skillet with the cooked asparagus and stir to combine. Bake over low to medium heat until the eggs start bubbling.

6. Place the skillet in your oven and bake for about 15-20 minutes until the eggs are golden brown. Serve the dish warm.

Bacon Cheeseburger

Prep Time: 5 min

Cook Time: 15 min

Serve: 4

Ingredients:

- 1 lb. lean ground beef
- ¼ cup chopped yellow onion and 1 clove garlic, minced
- 1 Tbsp. yellow mustard
- 1 Tbsp. Worcestershire sauce
- ½ tsp salt Cooking spray
- 4 ultra-thin slices cheddar cheese, cut into 6 equal-sized rectangular pieces
- 3 pieces of turkey bacon, each cut into 8 evenly-sized rectangular pieces
- 24 dill pickle chips 4-6 green leaf

- lettuce leaves, torn into 24 small square-shaped pieces 12 cherry tomatoes, sliced in half

Directions:

1. Pre-heat oven to 400°F. Combine the garlic, salt, onion, Worcestershire sauce, and beef in a medium-sized bowl, and mix well. Form mixture into 24 small meatballs. Put meatballs onto a foil- lined baking sheet and cook for 12-15 minutes. Leave oven on.

2. Top every meatball with a piece of cheese, then go back to the oven until cheese melts for about 2 to 3 minutes. Let meatballs cool.

3. To assemble bites: on a toothpick layer a cheese-covered meatball, piece of bacon, piece of lettuce, pickle chip, and a tomato half.

Cheeseburger Pie

Prep Time: 25 min

Cook Time: 90 min

Serve: 4

Ingredients:

- 1 large spaghetti squash
- 1 lb. lean ground beef
- ¼ cup diced onion
- 2 eggs
- 1/3 cup low-fat, plain Greek yogurt
- 2 Tbsp. Tomato sauce
- ½ tsp Worcestershire sauce
- 2/3 cup reduced-fat, shredded cheddar cheese
- 2 oz dill pickle slices
- Cooking spray

Directions:

1. Preheat oven to 400°F. Slice spaghetti squash in half lengthwise; dismiss pulp and seeds. Spray cooking spray.

2. Place the cut pumpkin halves on a foil-lined baking sheet and bake for 30 minutes. Once cooked, let it cool before scraping the pulp from the squash with a fork to remove the spaghetti-like strings. set aside.

3. Push squash strands in the bottom and up sides of the greased pie pan, creating an even layer.

4. Meanwhile, set up pie filling. In a lightly greased, medium-sized skillet, cook beef and onion over medium heat 8 to 10 minutes, sometimes stirring, until meat is brown. Drain and remove from heat.

5. The eggs, tomato paste, Greek yogurt and Worcestershire sauce and add the ground beef mixture. Pour the pie filling over the pumpkin

rind. Sprinkle the meat filling with cheese, then fill with pickled cucumber slices.

6. Bake for 40 minutes.

Ancho Tilapia
On Cauliflower Rice

Prep Time: 15 min

Cook Time: 30 min

Serve: 4

Ingredients:

- 2 lbs. tilapia
- 1 tsp lime juice
- 1 tsp salt
- 1 tbsp ground ancho pepper
- 1 tsp ground cumin
- 1 ½ tbsp. extra virgin olive oil
- ¼ cup toasted pumpkin seeds
- 6 cups cauliflower rice minutes
- 1 cup coarsely chopped fresh cilantro

Directions:

1. Preheat oven to 450°F. Dress tilapia with lime juice and set aside. Combine cumin, ancho pepper, and salt in a bowl. Season tilapia with spice mixture.

2. Lay tilapia on a baking sheet or casserole dish and bake for 7 minutes. In the meantime, in a big skillet, sweat the cauliflower rice in olive oil till tender, about 2-3 minutes.

3. Blend the pumpkin seeds and cilantro into the rice. Dismiss from heat, and serve.

Eggs with Zucchini Noodles

Prep Time: 10 min

Cook Time: 11 min

Serve: 2

Ingredients:

- 2 tablespoons extra-virgin olive oil
- 3 zucchinis, cut with a spiralizer
- 4 eggs
- Salt and black pepper to the taste
- A pinch of red pepper flakes
- Cooking spray
- 1 tablespoon basil, chopped

Directions:

1. In a bowl, combine the zucchini noodles with salt, pepper and the olive oil and toss well.

2. Grease a baking sheet with your cooking spray and divide the zucchini noodles into 4 nests on it.

3. Crack an egg on top of every nest, sprinkle salt, pepper and the pepper flakes on top, bake at 350 degrees F for 11 minutes.

4. Divide the mix between plates, sprinkle the basil on top and serve.

Banana Oats

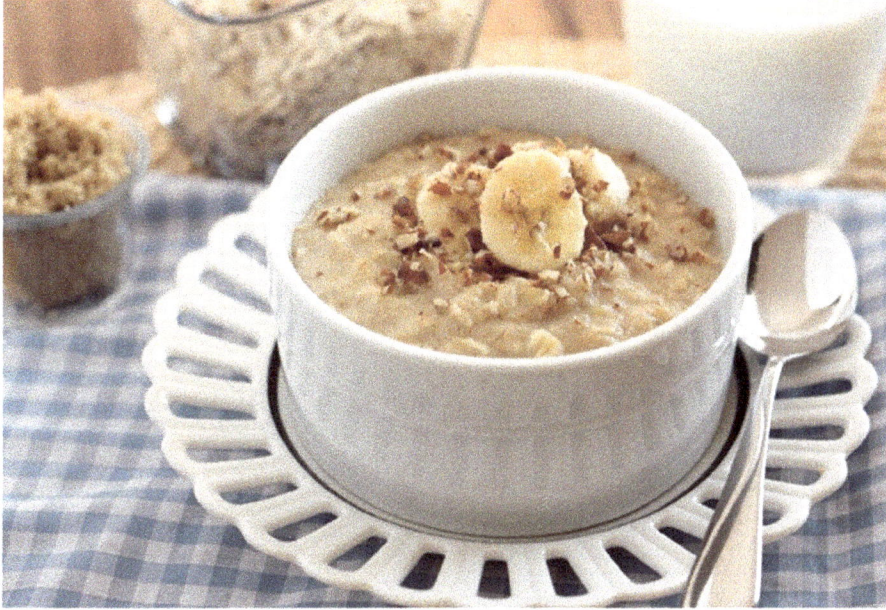

Prep Time: 10 min

Cook Time: 0 min

Serve: 2

Ingredients:

- 1 banana, peeled and sliced
- ¾ cup almond milk
- ½ cup cold brewed coffee
- 2 dates, pitted
- 2 tablespoons cocoa powder

- 1 cup rolled oats
- 1 and ½ tablespoons chia seeds

Directions:

1. In a blender, combine the banana with the milk and the rest of the ingredients, pulse, divide into bowls, and serve breakfast.

Slow-cooked Peppers Frittata

Prep Time: 10 min

Cook time: 3 h

Serve: 6

Ingredients:

- ½ cup almond milk
- 8 eggs, whisked
- Salt and pepper to the taste
- 1 teaspoon oregano, dried
- 1 and ½ cups roasted peppers, chopped
- ½ cup red onion, chopped
- 4 cups baby arugula
- 1 cup goat cheese, crumbled
- Cooking spray

Directions:

1. In a bowl, combine the eggs with salt, pepper and the oregano and whisk.

2. Grease your slow cooker with the cooking spray, arrange the peppers and the remaining ingredients, and pour the eggs mixture over them.

3. Put the lid on and then cook on Low for 3 hours. Divide the frittata between plates and serve.

Apple Quinoa Bowl

Prep Time: 10 min

Cook Time: 15 min

Serve: 2

Ingredients:

- ½ Cup Quinoa, Uncooked
- 1 Cup Vanilla Almond Milk, Unsweetened
- ½ Teaspoon Cinnamon
- 2 Cinnamon Sticks
- Pinch Sea Salt Toppings:
- 2 Tablespoons Almonds, Sliced
- 2 Tablespoons Hemp Seeds
- Cup Apple, Chopped Honey to Sweeten

Preparation:

1. Rinse your quinoa using a colander and make sure it's well drained. Transfer it to a saucepan with your cinnamon, cinnamon sticks, almond milk and salt. Bring it to a simmer, and cover.

Reduce to low, allowing it to simmer for fifteen minutes.

2. Remove it from heat and then let it rest for five minutes. 3. Your almond milk should be absorbed, and you should cook your quinoa all the way through.

4. Divide between bowls and top with your toppings.

Overnight Chia Pudding

Prep Time: 8 h and 5 min

Cook Time: 0 min

Serve: 2

Ingredients:

- ½ Cup Chia Seeds
- 2n Cups Coconut Milk, Light
- 3 Teaspoons Honey, Divided
- ¼ Cup Banana, Sliced
- ¼ Cup Raspberries, Fresh
- ½ Tablespoon Almonds, Sliced
- ½ Tablespoon Walnuts, Chopped
- 2 Teaspoons Cocoa Powder, Unsweetened & Divided
-

Preparation:

1. Mix your chia seeds, coconut milk, and two teaspoons of honey in a bowl. Portion it out into

mason jars, and refrigerate for eight hours or overnight.

2. Remove them from the fridge, and top with raspberries, almonds, banana, cocoa and walnuts. Drizzle with remaining honey.

Avocado Toast

Prep Time: 10 min

Cook Time: 0 min

Serve: 2

Ingredients:

- 1 tablespoon goat cheese, crumbled
- 1 avocado, peeled, pitted and mashed
- A pinch of salt and black pepper
- 2 whole wheat bread slices, toasted
- ½ teaspoon lime juice
- 1 persimmon, thinly sliced
- 1 fennel bulb, thinly sliced 2 teaspoons honey
- 2 tablespoons pomegranate seeds
-

Preparation:

1. In a bowl, combine the avocado with salt, pepper, lime juice and the cheese and whisk.

2. Spread this onto toasted bread slices, top each slice with the remaining ingredients and serve for breakfast.

Green Juice

Prep Time: 5 min

Serve: 1

Ingredients:

- 1/4 cup fresh Italian parsley leaves
- 1/4 sliced pineapple
- 1/2 green apple
- 1/2 lemon
- 1/2 orange
- A pinch of grated fresh ginger
-

Preparation:

Use a juicer to run the greens cucumber parsley pineapple apple orange lemon and ginger through it pour into a large cup and serve.

Healthy Chocolate Banana Smoothie

Prep Time: 5 min

Serve: 2

Ingredients:

- 2 bananas
- 4 ice cubes (if you don't have frozen banana)
- 1 cup unsweetened almond milk or skim milk
- 1 cup crushed ice
- 3 tablespoons unsweetened cocoa powder (to taste)
- 3 tablespoons sugar or honey

Preparation:

In a blender jar pour milk and add banana almond milk ice cocoa powder and honey. Blend until smooth.

Fruit Smoothie

Prep Time: 5 min

Serve: 2

Ingredients:

- 2 cups blueberries
- 2 cups unsweetened almond milk
- 1 cup crushed ice
- 1/2 teaspoon ground ginger

Preparation:

Combine the blueberries almond milk ice and ginger in a blender. Blend until smooth.

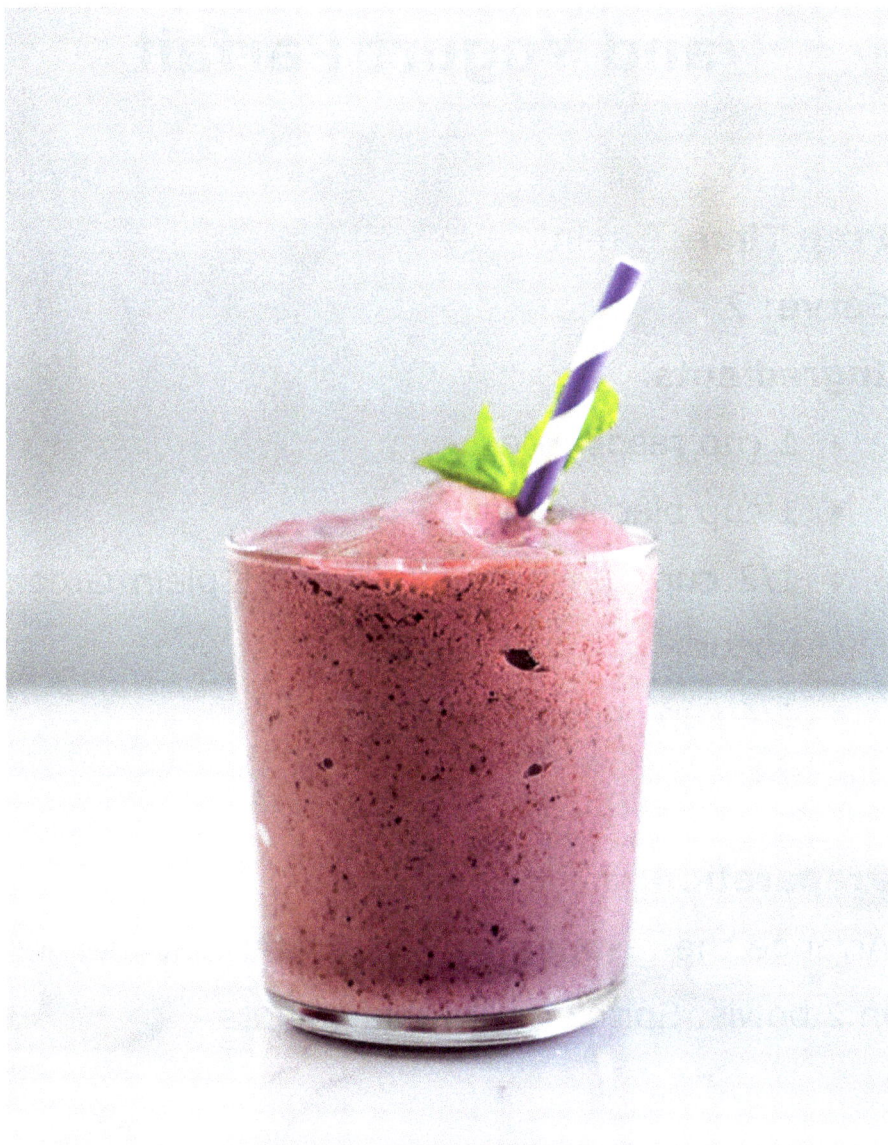

Mixed Berry
and Yogurt Parfait

Prep Time: 5 min

Serve: 2

Ingredients:

- 1 cup raspberries
- 1 cup blackberries
- 1/2 cups unsweetened nonfat plain Greek yogurt
- 1/4 cup chopped walnuts

Preparation:

Arrange the raspberries yogurt and blackberries in 2 bowls. Sprinkle with the walnuts.

Yogurt Blueberries Honey and Mint Combination

Prep Time: 5 min

Serve: 2

Ingredients:

- 2 cups unsweetened nonfat plain Greek yogurt
- 1 cup blueberries
- 3 tablespoons honey
- 2 tablespoons fresh mint leaves chopped
-

Preparation:

Share out the yogurt between 2 small bowls. Top with the blueberries honey and mint.

Almond and Maple Quick Grits

Prep Time: 5 min

Cook Time: 6 min

Serve: 4

Ingredients:

- 11/2 cups water
- 1/2 cup unsweetened almond milk
- Pinch sea salt
- 1/2 cup quick-cooking grits
- 1/2 teaspoon ground cinnamon
- 1/4 cup pure maple syrup
- 1/4 cup slivered almonds

Preparation:

1. Heat the water almond milk and sea salt in a medium saucepan over medium-high heat until it boils.

2. Stirring constantly with a spoon and slowly add the grits. Continue stirring to prevent lumps and bring the mixture to a slow boil. Reduce the heat to medium-low.

3. Simmer for 6 minutes stirring frequently, continue till the water is completely absorbed. Add the cinnamon syrup and almonds while you stir.

4. Cook for 1 minute more and stir.

Oatmeal Topped with Berries and Sunflower Seeds

Prep Time: 15 min

Serve: 4

Ingredients:

- 13/4 cups water
- 1/2 clip unsweetened almond milk
- 1 cup old-fashioned oats
- 1/2 cup blueberries
- 1/2 cup raspberries
- 1/4 cup sunflower seeds
- A pinch of sea salt

Preparation:

1. In a saucepan over medium-high heat, then heat the almond milk and sea salt to a boil.

2. Gently pour in the oat as you stir. Reduce the heat and cook for 5 - 6 minutes.

3. Cover and let the oatmeal stand for 2 minutes more. Stir and serve topped with the blueberries raspberries and sunflower seeds.

Eggy Bread

Prep Time: 30 min

Serve: 6

Ingredients:

- 6 light whole-wheat bread slices
- 11/2 clips unsweetened almond milk
- 2 eggs beaten
- 2 egg whites beaten
- 1 teaspoon vanilla extract
- Zest of 1 orange
- Juice of 1 orange
- 1 teaspoon ground nutmeg
- Nonstick cooking spray

Preparation:

1. Using a shallow bowl whisk the almond milk, eggs, egg whites, vanilla, orange zest and juice and nutmeg.

2. Place the bread in one single layer in a 9-by-13-inch baking dish. Pour the milk and egg mixture over the top. Allow the bread to soak for about few minutes turning once.

3. Spray a nonstick skillet with cooking spray and heat over medium-high heat. Working in batches add the bread and then cook for about 5 minutes per side until the custard sets.

Zucchini-Tomato Frittata

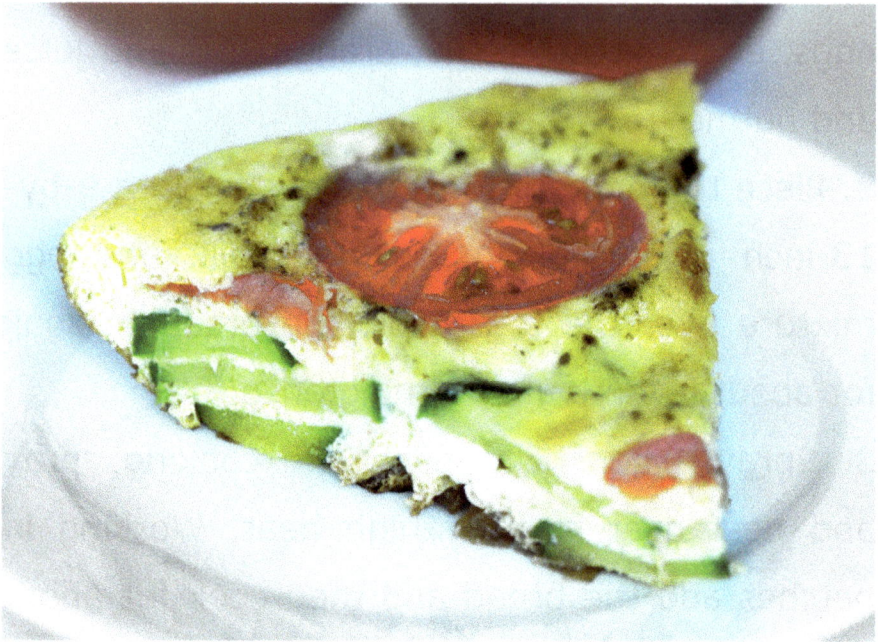

Prep Time: 10 min

Cook time: 8 min

Serve: 4

Ingredients:

- 3 eggs
- 3 egg whites
- 1/2 cup unsweetened almond
- milk

- 1/2 teaspoon sea salt
- Vs teaspoon freshly ground black pepper
- 2 tablespoons extra-virgin olive oil
- 1 zucchini chopped
- 8 cherry tomatoes halved
- 1/4 cup (about 2 ounces) grated Parmesan cheese

Preparation:

1. Preheat the oven's broiler to high temperature of about 400'F adjusting the oven rack to the center position.

2. Vigorously whisk the eggs egg whites almond milk sea salt and pepper in a shallow bowel. Set aside.

3. In an about 12-inch ovenproof skillet heat the olive oil until it shimmers. Now add the zucchini and tomatoes and cook for 5 minutes stirring occasionally. Pour the egg cream over the vegetables and cook for about 4 minutes

without stirring until the eggs set around the edges.

4. Using a silicone spatula pull the set eggs away from the edges of the pan. Tilt the pan in all directions to allow the unset eggs to fill the spaces along the edges. Cook for about 4 minutes more without stirring until the edges set again.

5. Apply the eggs with the Parmesan. Transfer the pan to the broiler. Cook until the cheese melts and your eggs are puffy about 3 to 5 minutes. Cut into wedges to serve.

Scramble Egg with Smoked Salmon

Prep Time: 5 min

Cook time: 10 min

Serve: 4

Ingredients:

- 4 eggs
- 6 egg whites
- 1/8 teaspoon freshly ground black pepper
- 2 tablespoons extra-virgin olive
- oil
- 1/2 red onion finely chopped and 4 ounces smoked salmon flaked
- 2 tablespoons capers drained

Preparation:

1. In a small bowl whisk the eggs whites and pepper. Set aside. In a large nonstick skillet heat the olive oil until it shimmers.

2. Add the onion and let cook for about 3 minutes while stirring until soft. Cook the salmon and capers together for 1 minute.

3. Cook the egg mixture in a pan for about 3 to 5 minutes stirring frequently or until the eggs are set.

Poached Eggs with Avocado Toast

Prep Time: 10 min

Cook time: 5 min

Serve: 4

Ingredients:

- 2 avocados peeled and pitted
- 1/4 cup chopped fresh basil leaves
- 3 tablespoons red swine vinegar divided
- Juice of 1 lemon
- Zest of 1 lemon
- 1 garlic clove minced
- 1 teaspoon sea salt divided
- 1/8 teaspoon freshly ground black pepper
- Pinch cayenne pepper plus more as needed
- 4 eggs

Preparation:

1. In a blender combine the avocados basil 2 tablespoons of vinegar the lemon juice and zest garlic 1/2 teaspoon of sea salt pepper and cayenne. Purée for about 1 minute until smooth.

2. Fill a 12-inch nonstick skillet about three-fourths full of water and place it over medium heat. Add the residual tablespoon of vinegar and the remaining 1/2 teaspoon of sea salt. Bring the water to a simmer.

3. Carefully crack the eggs into custard cups. Holding the cups just barely above the water carefully slip theeggs into the simmering water one at a time. Turn off the heat and then cover the skillet. Let the eggs sit for 5 minutes without agitating the pan or removing the lid.

4. Using a slotted spoon carefully lift the eggs from the water allowing them to drain completely. Place each egg on a plate and spoon the avocado purée over the top.

Poached Pears

Prep Time: 15 min

Cook Time: 30 min

Serve: 4

Ingredients:

- 4 Pears, Whole
- ¼ Cup Apple Juice
- 1 Cup Orange Juice
- 1 Teaspoon Cinnamon
- 1 Teaspoon Nutmeg
- ½ Cup Raspberries, Fresh
- 2 Tablespoons Orange Zest
-

Preparation:

1. Combine your apple juice, orange juice, nutmeg and cinnamon in a bowl. Peel your pears and make sure to leave the stems on.

Remove the core, but make sure to remove them from the bottom.

2. Combine your juices and pears in a shallow pan. Cook over medium heat, and bring it to a simmer.

3. Allow it to simmer for a half hour. Turn them regularly, making sure they don't come to a boil. Garnish with orange zest and raspberries.

Marinated Berries

Prep Time: 2 h 15 min

Cook Time: 0 min

Serve: 2

Ingredients:

- ¼ Cup Balsamic Vinegar
- ½ Cup Strawberries
- ½ Cup Blueberries
- ½ Cup Raspberries
- 2 Shortbread Biscuits
- 2 Tablespoons Brown Sugar and 1 Teaspoon Vanilla Extract, Pure

Preparation:

1. Start by mixing your brown sugar, vanilla and balsamic vinegar in a bowl, and then blend your berries in another bowl. Pour your marinade on top of the fruit, and allow it to marinate for ten to fifteen minutes.

2. Drain, and then allow it to chill for up to two hours.

3. Distribute the chilled fruit in bowls served with shortbread on the side.

Cannellini Bean Soup

Prep Time: 5 min

Cook Time: 20 min

Serve: 4

Ingredients:

- Two sliced potatoes
- 2 cups vegetable broth
- Two cans of cannellini beans
- 1-2 diced garlic cloves
- 1/8 tsp pepper and 1/3 cup white wine
- 1/2 tsp paprika
- 1/2 tsp salt
- 1 tbsp tomato paste
- 1 tbsp of olive oil
- One sprig rosemary
- One diced onion
- One diced carrot
- 1 cup spinach
- One diced celery stalk

Preparation:

1. Heat the oil in a big kettle. Add the diced celery, carrot, and onion until the oil shimmers. Cook for 5 minutes, stirring until the onion is soft and turns translucent.

2. Add the potatoes, tomato paste, beans, garlic, rosemary (whatever is better for you, the whole sprig, sliced, or dried), and paprika. (if you use it). (if you use it). (if you use it). (if you use it). (if you use it). (if you use it). Cook for about 1 minute, stirring constantly.

3. Pour in the wine, mix well, and let it boil for another minute until it has evaporated. Then include frozen spinach in the vegetables' broth and a pleasant pinch of salt & pepper. Boost the heat, boil the mixture, gently cover the kettle, and reduce the heat and simmer for 15 minutes.

4. Remove the pot from the heat until the potatoes are soft and the soup is dense and fluffy, then remove the rosemary sprig*. Taste

and season with pepper and salt. Based on the vegetable broth or your preferences, you can need more salt.

5. Break into cups, drizzle with extra virgin olive oil or olive oil, and add more ground black pepper as you prefer. Serve with the crusty whole-grain bread, and add fresh parmesan cheese for extra spice if you do not keep it vegan. Enjoy!

Garlic, sweet potato, and chickpea soup

Prep Time: 10 min

Cook time: 30 min

Serve: 4-6

Ingredients:

- lemon juice
- Eight cloves garlic, sliced
- 400 g chickpeas
- 350 g cooked sweet potato
- 30 g olive oil
- 2 tsp ground turmeric
- 2 tsp dried thyme
- 1 tsp salt
- One chopped onion
- ½ tsp cayenne pepper

Preparation:

1. In a big saucepan with water, place the garlic, olive oil, and onions: this produces more steam to rapidly tender the garlic. Then bring the fire to a boil and simmer for five min until the water evaporates and the garlic is very tender.

2. Add the sweet potatoes, salt, thyme, turmeric, chickpeas, cayenne, and 800 ml of water, and bring to a boil until the sweet potatoes have further softened. Remove from the sun and slightly cool off.

3. In a mixer, puree the mixture until creamy. If necessary, return to the pan, change the consistency with additional water, and then heat it until it boils. Divide between 4 and 6 bowls and apply a drizzle of lemon juice and a few shreds of black pepper to each bowl.

Kumara, coconut, and lemongrass soup

Prep Time: 10 min

Cook Time: 25 min

Serve: 6

Ingredients:

- One chopper White onion
- 5 cups of Vegetable Stock Thai Basil - for garnish
- 2 lb chopped Sweet Potatoes
- 2 tbsp Olive Oil
- 2 Lemongrass Stalks
- 2 Kaffir Lime Leaves
- ½ tsp chopped ginger
- ½ tbsp Chopped garlic
- ½ cup Coconut Milk
- Four chopped Celery Stalks

Preparation:

1. On a moderate flame, heat the olive oil. Sweat until the onion is transparent, the chopped onion, ginger, lemongrass, garlic, lime leaves, and celery.

2. Add in the vegetable supply and sweet potatoes. Carry to a boil, reduce the heat until it is cooked and then simmer cover for around 25 min or until the sweet potatoes are softened.

3. Now give a minute for the soup to cool off. Please cut the lime leaves and the lemongrass before you mix it into a smooth broth. Move all the ingredients carefully into your blender or cream the soup with a handheld blender.

4. Put the soup back in a clean dish, reheat, and add the milk from the coconut. Taste the broth and season with white pepper and some salt, if possible. Reheat the soup before eating, put it in bowls, and spread some Thai basil on top.

Moroccan Chickpea Soup

Prep Time: 15 min

Cook Time: 30 min

Serve: 3

Ingredients:

- coriander sprigs
- 500 ml of vegetable stock
- 40 g seed mix, roasted
- 410 g tin chickpeas
- 400 g chopped tomatoes
- 1 tsp cumin seeds
- 1 tbsp olive oil
- One chopped red pepper
- One chopped onion
- One crushed garlic clove
- One chopped carrot

Preparation:

Heat the olive oil in a saucepan, then add the seeds of onion, carrot, garlic, pepper, and cumin and fry for around 5 minutes. Stir in the stock and the tomatoes, and cook for 5 minutes. Using a hand blender to purée the onions, stir in chickpeas, and heat them for 2 minutes. Adorn with coriander/beans. With bread, serve.

Creamy and rich Spicy Pumpkin

Prep Time: 5 min

Cook Time: 25 min

Serve: 1/4

Ingredients:

- 1 cup milk
- 15 oz pumpkin puree
- One clove garlic, minced
- One onion, chopped
- 1/2 tsp Cajun seasoning
- 1/4 tbsp heavy cream
- 1/4 tsp crushed red pepper
- 2 1/2 cups chicken broth
- 2 tbsp brown sugar
- 2 tbsp butter Pepitas, for serving
- Pinch of cayenne pepper

1. Over the medium-high heat, heat the butter in the big saucepan either in a Dutch oven.

Preparation:

1. Add the onion and simmer for about 4 minutes, constantly stirring, until tender. Apply the garlic and then cook for an extra thirty seconds. Apply the Cajun, cayenne

pepper, and red pepper. Season and steam for another 30 seconds.

2. Add a pumpkin puree and broth with the chicken. Until smooth, stir. Bring to boil, then simmer for 10-15 mins and reduce the heat. Move the soup to a mixer or food processor, in batches. Tightly cover and mix until smooth. Set the soup back in the dish.

3. Add brown sugar and whisk until melted, when the heat is low. Add in the milk gently, and stir constantly. Taste, then change the

taste of the seasonings. If required, finish each serving with tablespoons of cream and pepitas.

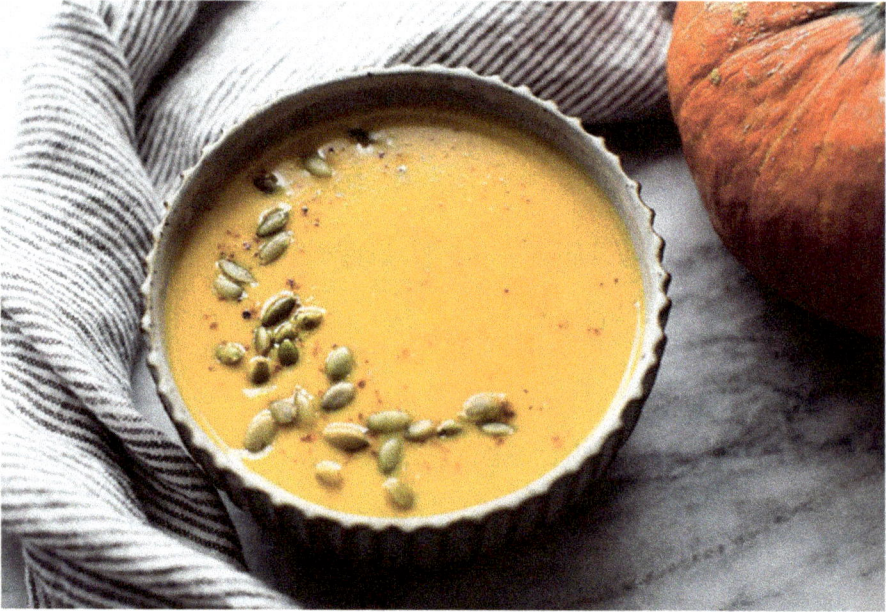

Ribollita

Prep Time: 15 min

Cook Time: 25 min

Serve: 10

Ingredients:

- 1 1/2 tsp salt
- 14 oz crushed tomatoes
- One red onion, chopped
- 1 lb chopped cavolo nero
- 1/2 lb loaf of bread
- Two chopped carrots
- Three cloves garlic, chopped
- 3 tbsp olive oil
- Four celery stalks, chopped
- 4 cups white beans, cooked chopped black olives
- 1/2 tsp of red pepper flakes zest of one lemon

Preparation:

1. Mix the olive oil, garlic, carrot, celery, and red onion in the largest dense pot over medium heat. Sweat the vegetables for 10 -15 minutes, but stop further browning. Add the tomatoes and flakes of red pepper and cook for another ten minutes, long enough to make the tomatoes thicken a little. Add the cavolo nero, and 8 cups of water, 3 cups of beans, per 2 liters. Bring it to a boil, reduce the heat and cook for around 15 minutes until the greens are tender.

2. Meanwhile, with a generous splash of water, mash or puree the remaining beans - till smooth. Tear the bread into chunks. Add the bread and the beans to the soup. Simmer, stirring regularly, for 20 minutes or so, before the bread disintegrates and the soup becomes thick. Add the salt, taste and if appropriate, add more. Stir in the zest of the lemon.

3. Serve instantly, or cool overnight and refrigerate. With a bit of olive oil and some chopped olives, finish each serving.

Broccoli soup

Prep Time: 10 min

Cook Time: 25 min

Serve: 6

Ingredients:

- One onion, chopped
- One stalk celery, chopped
- 2 cups of milk
- 3 cups chicken brot
- 3 tbsp all-purpose flour and 5 tbsp butter
- 8 cups broccoli florets black pepper to taste

Preparation:

1. In a medium-sized stock container, heat two tablespoons of butter and sauté the celery and onion until tender. Add the broccoli and broth, then cover for 10 minutes and simmer.

2. In a mixer, pour the broth, filling the pitcher but no more than halfway full. With the folded kitchen towel, keep the blender's lid down and start the blender carefully, using a few short pulses to transfer the soup before leaving it to puree. Purée until smooth and dump into a clean pot in batches. Alternately, right in the frying pot, you should use a stick blender to puree the broth.

3. Melt three tablespoons of butter in a shallow saucepan, whisk in the flour and add the cream. Stir until bubbly and thick, and apply to the broth. Season and eat with pepper.

Mushroom soup

Prep Time: 5 min

Cook Time: 45 min

Serve: 6

Ingredients:

- Salt to taste
- Black pepper to taste
- Six sprigs thyme
- 4 cups chicken stock
- 3 tbsp olive oil
- 1/4 cup whipping cream
- 1/4 cup Cognac
- 1/4 cup chopped chives
- 1/2 cup minced shallot
- One sprig rosemary
- 1 lb mixed mushrooms
- 1 lb cremini mushrooms

Preparation:

1. Chop the mushroom stems roughly and let them simmer and covered for about an hour in the chicken broth. In a large skillet, heat the oil and sauté each shallot until they are transparent. Lightly add the spices, salt, and pepper.

2. Chop the mushroom caps beautifully and precisely into the 1/2-inch dice. Add them as they are sliced into the shallots. Keep the heat very low until the mushroom fluid is released and then reabsorbed, and cook gently. Shake the cup so that they do not stick. Remove the rosemary and thyme. Turn the heat up, then add the Cognac.

3. Flame it up if you just feel like Chef-y. Cook down the mushroom cap or shallot mixture until well-reduced and begin to turn the edges a bit golden.

4. Strain the fungus from the broth of the chicken. To the filtered broth, apply the wonderful shallot mixture and mushroom cap

and heat it gently. Swirl in and serve the cream and chives. Or serve, if you like to get fancy, in tiny sipping bowls topped with chives and softly whipped cream.

Chickpea & Pomegranate Dip

Prep Time: 10 min

Cook Time: 0 min

Serve: 5

Ingredients:

- 3 tbsp pomegranate molasses
- 2 tbsp chopped mint
- 2 tbsp chopped coriander
- 12 oz chickpeas
- 1/4 cup of red Onion
- 1/4 cup crumbled feta cheese
- 1/2 tsp salt
- 1/2 tsp hot pepper flakes
- 1/2 cup olive oil
- One clove garlic minced
- 1 tsp ground cumin

Preparation:

1. Put pulse chickpeas, pomegranate molasses, oil, all but one teaspoon (about 5 mL) both of the mint & coriander along with cumin, salt, and pepper flakes together in the food processor until mixed, but still a little bit chunky.

2. Onion pulse; whisk in garlic. Scrap the serving bowl into it. (Make- ahead: Up to 24 hours to cover and refrigerate.) Dust with feta and leftover mint and coriander.

Guacamole

Prep Time: 10 min

Cook Time: 10 min

Serve: 4

Ingredients:

- ½ cup diced Onion
- One lime, juiced
- One pinch of cayenne pepper
- 1 tsp minced garlic
- 1 tsp salt
- 2 Roma tomatoes, diced
- Three mashed avocados
- 3 tbsp chopped cilantro

Preparation:

Mash the avocados along with lime juice and salt in a medium cup. Combine the cilantro, tomato, onion, and garlic. Stir in the pepper with cayenne. For the best taste, refrigerate for 1 hour or serve it immediately.

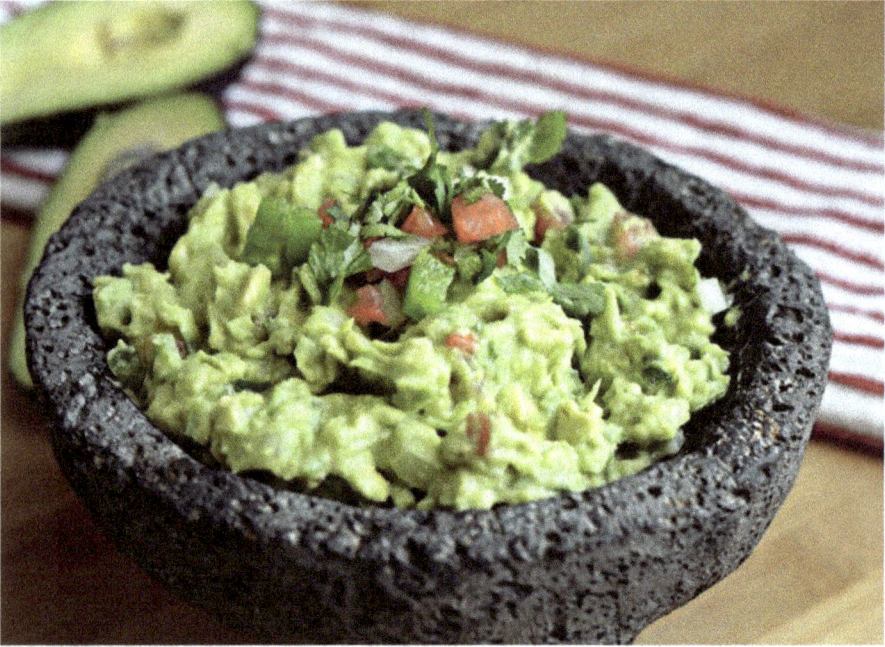

www.ingramcontent.com/pod-product-compliance
Lightning Source LLC
Chambersburg PA
CBHW050754030426
42336CB00012B/1808